80 Gallbladder Stone Preventing Meal and Juice Recipes:

Using Proper Dieting and Smart Nutritional Habits to Reduce Your Chances of Developing Gall Bladder Stones

By

Joe Correa CSN

COPYRIGHT

This publication is designed to provide accurate and authoritative information in regard to the subject matter covered. It is sold with the understanding that neither the author nor the publisher is engaged in rendering medical advice. If medical advice or assistance is needed, consult with a doctor. This book is considered a guide and should not be used in any way detrimental to your health. Consult with a physician before starting this nutritional plan to make sure it's right for you.

ACKNOWLEDGEMENTS

This book is dedicated to my friends and family that have had mild or serious illnesses so that you may find a solution and make the necessary changes in your life.

80 Gallbladder Stone Preventing Meal and Juice Recipes:

Using Proper Dieting and Smart Nutritional Habits to Reduce Your Chances of Developing Gall Bladder Stones

By

Joe Correa CSN

CONTENTS

ABOUT THE AUTHOR

After years of Research, I honestly believe in the positive effects that proper nutrition can have over the body and mind. My knowledge and experience has helped me live healthier throughout the years and which I have shared with family and friends. The more you know about eating and drinking healthier, the sooner you will want to change your life and eating habits.

Nutrition is a key part in the process of being healthy and living longer so get started today. The first step is the most important and the most significant.

INTRODUCTION

80 Gallbladder Stone Preventing Meal and Juice Recipes: Using Proper Dieting and Smart Nutritional Habits to Reduce Your Chances of Developing Gall Bladder Stones

By Joe Correa CSN

Gallstones develop when the bile becomes overly concentrated with cholesterol forming crystals that become hard stones in the gallbladder. A healthy bile and a healthy bile flow are essential in order to prevent gallstone formation.

The worst things for your bile are foods that are high in fat, cholesterol, refined carbohydrates, saturated fats present in processed, fried, and fatty red meat and should be avoided at all costs. Make sure your diet is high in fiber.

In order to promote a healthy bile and bile flow a diet rich in fruits, vegetables, lean meats, low-fat dairy products and whole-grain foods should be a part of your well-balanced diet.

The recipes in this book will help you prevent and treat gallstones. Use these recipes every day to help you to have a healthy gallbladder and live a longer life. The meal and juices recipes in this book are full of fiber and nutrient-rich foods that will make a big difference in your diet. Get started today!

80 GALLBLADDER STONE PREVENTING MEAL AND JUICE RECIPES: USING PROPER DIETING AND SMART NUTRITIONAL HABITS TO REDUCE YOUR CHANCES OF DEVELOPING GALL BLADDER STONES

MEALS

1.   Fruity Breakfast yogurt

A diet that is high in fat, especially full-fat dairy should be avoided. Eating foods high in cholesterol or in fat can increased blood cholesterol levels. If the gallbladder does not make enough bile to dissolve the cholesterol, this cholesterol may form into gallstones.

Ingredients:

1 cup Yogurt, plain

1 Tbsp. Strawberry

1 Tbsp. Mango

½ Banana, thinly sliced

1 Tbsp. Dried pears, cut into small pieces

2 Tbsp. Corn flakes

Preparation:

Stir all contents in one bowl. Serve chilled. Enjoy for breakfast!

Serving Size 427 g

Amount per Serving

Calories 449

Calories from Fat 41

Total Fat 4.5g

Saturated Fat 2.8g

Cholesterol 15mg

Sodium 209mg

Potassium 1378mg

Total Carbohydrates 86.0g

Dietary Fiber 7.2g

Sugars 72.1g

Protein 17.7g

Vitamin A 37% • Vitamin C 117% • Calcium 47% • Iron 8%

2. Steamed fish with broccoli

Consuming a diet low in cholesterol and calories reduces the risk of gallstones. Vegetables such as broccoli are rich in fiber which is essential in preventing gallstones.

Ingredients:

1 lb. Broccoli, rinsed and cut into small pieces

2 fillet Snapper

1 tsp. Lemon juice

1 Tbsp. Green onion

1 tsp. Garlic

1 tsp. Salt

1/8 tsp. Pepper

2 Tbsp. Olive oil

Preparation:

Place the broccoli in a microwave-safe bowl with 3 tablespoons of water. Cover with a lid and microwave for 3-4 minutes or until leaves are brilliant emerald green. Season with a pinch of salt and pepper.

Rub the snapper fillet with olive oil, garlic, salt and pepper. Drizzle with lemon juice. Sprinkle with green onion.

Transfer to a microwave-safe dish. Cover with a lid and place it in the microwave for 4-5 minutes depending on the thickness the fillets.

Serving Size 252 g

Amount Per Serving

Calories 201

Calories from Fat 133

Total Fat 14.8g

Saturated Fat 2.0g

Trans Fat 0.0g

Cholesterol 0mg

Sodium 1239mg

Potassium 737mg

Total Carbohydrates 15.9g

Dietary Fiber 6.1g

Sugars 4.0g

Protein 6.5g

Vitamin A 29% • Vitamin C 341%• %Calcium 11%•Iron 10%

3. Raw shredded beet salad

Beets strengthen the bladder walls and cleanses the gallbladder. It also cleanses the colon and blood, and thins the consistency of the bile making it flow smoothly. It metabolizes fats and relieves symptoms of a gallbladder attack.

Ingredients:

4 pcs. Beetroots, scrubbed, peeled and shredded

1 large Potato, boiled, peeled and cubed into 1"

1 large Shallots, minced

1 Tbsp. Mustard

1 Tbsp. Extra virgin olive oil

1 Tbsp. Parsley, minced

Preparation:

Toss everything in a bowl, mix and serve.

Serving Size 200 g

Amount Per Serving

Calories 229

Calories from Fat 79

Total Fat 8.8g

Saturated Fat 1.1g

Cholesterol 0mg

Sodium 12mg

Potassium 825mg

Total Carbohydrates 34.3g

Dietary Fiber 4.9g

Sugars 1.8g

Protein 5.2g

Vitamin A 3% • Vitamin C 65%• %Calcium 5%•Iron 12%

4.   Classic veggie wrap

Cucumber contains high amount of water which is ideal for detoxifying the gallbladder. Carrots are a good source of vitamin C and is rich in other nutrients. Recent research shows that vitamin C helps convert cholesterol to bile acids reducing cholesterol crystallization or gallstones formation.

Ingredients:

½ cup Cucumbers, cubed

1 Tomatoes, chopped

1 Onion, chopped

1 Carrot, shredded

6 Tbsp. Fat-free greek yogurt

1 Tbsp. Dijon mustard

2 Whole wheat tortillas

Preparation:

In a small bowl combine the yogurt and mustard. Slather on wrap. Add all vegies and roll wrap.

Serving Size 228 g

Amount Per Serving

Calories 165

Calories from Fat 14

Total Fat 1.5g

Trans Fat 0.0g

Cholesterol 0mg

Sodium 245mg

Potassium 373mg

Total Carbohydrates 33.9g

Dietary Fiber 6.1g

Sugars 6.0g

Protein 5.9g

Vitamin A 113% • Vitamin C 25% • Calcium 8% • Iron 9%

5.   Green beans with shitake mushroom in lemon garlic sauce

Green beans contain high amount of fiber which is beneficial in improving intestinal health, preventing heart disease and certain cancers, regulating blood sugar and lowering of cholesterol level in the body.

Ingredients:

3 cups Green beans, cut into 1"

2 Tbsp. Garlic

½ cup Shallots, thinly sliced

½ cup Shitake mushrooms, sliced thinly

¼ cup Olive oil

2 Tbsp. Lemon juice

1/8 tsp. Salt

1/8 tsp. Pepper

Preparation:

Over medium heat, heat the olive oil and stir in the garlic, shallots, shitake mushrooms and green beans. Stir-fry for 3 minutes or until garlic and shallots are brown and tender. Add the lemon juice and season with salt and pepper. Remove from heat, transfer to a plate and enjoy!

Serving Size 292 g

Amount Per Serving

Calories 332Calories from Fat 231

Total Fat 25.7g

Saturated Fat 3.8g

Cholesterol 0mg

Sodium 254mg

Potassium 575mg

Total Carbohydrates 26.7g

Dietary Fiber 6.6g

Sugars 4.0g

Protein 5.2g

Vitamin A 32% • Vitamin C 66% • Calcium 9% • Iron 14%

6.   Baked chicken with sweet potatoes

Sweet potatoes contain good carbohydrate that are loaded with fiber. The soluble fiber present in foods such as sweet potatoes slow down the passage of food through the intestines helping one feel full longer. It also helps lower the cholesterol level.

Ingredients:

3 pcs. Chicken breast fillet, butter-fly cut

3 Unpeeled medium sweet potatoes, scrubbed, rinsed and dried

3 tbsp. Olive oil

3 Tbsp. Sour cream

2 Tbsp. Green onion, chopped

1 tsp. Salt

1 tsp. Pepper

Boneless chicken breast marinade:

2 Tbsp. Balsamic vinegar

3 Tbsp. Oregano

2 Tbsp. Dijon mustard

¼ cup Shallots

¼ cup Olive oil

1/8 tsp. Salt

1/8 tsp. Pepper

Preparation:

In a bowl with lid, prepare the marinade by combining the balsamic vinegar, dijon mustard, shallots, olive oil, oregano, salt and pepper. Add the chicken breasts. Mix well. Cover with a lid and marinate overnight.

Preheat the oven to 350 F. Grease a baking tray with olive oil.

Pierce each potato with the tines of the fork 8 times, spacing evenly apart.

Place the marinated chicken and pierced sweet potatoes in a baking tray. Bake for 30 minutes or until chicken is thoroughly cooked. Remove chicken from the oven and transfer to a serving platter. Meanwhile, increase oven temperature to 400F. Continue baking the baked potato for another 10-15 minutes or until sweet potatoes are "fork-tender".

When potatoes are tender enough for a fork to be inserted without resistance, remove from the oven, cut into half and layer with sour cream. Season with salt and pepper. Top with green onions. Transfer to a serving platter together with the chicken.

Serving Size 135 g

Amount Per Serving

Calories 488

Calories from Fat 462

Total Fat 51.4g

Saturated Fat 9.2g

Trans Fat 0.0g

Cholesterol 8mg

Sodium 1503mg

Potassium 270mg

Total Carbohydrates 10.7g

Dietary Fiber 3.9g1

Sugars 0.7g

Protein 2.7g

Vitamin A 18% •Vitamin C 11% •Calcium 16%•Iron 22

7.   Stir-fried chicken with okra

Okra contains vitamin C, folic acid, calcium, and potassium. It is low in calories and contains high amount of dietary fiber. Okra has also been found to lower cholesterol levels.

Ingredients:

2 cups Okra, sliced in ¼ inches

1 cup Chicken breast, cubed

¾ cup Tomatoes

1/8 tsp. Turmeric powder

2 Tbsp. Garlic

1 Tbsp. Olive oil

1/8 tsp. Salt

1/8 tsp. Pepper

Preparation:

Over medium heat, saute garlic in olive oil until light brown. Stir in the tomatoes and okra. Cook until okra is tender and golden brown, or for about 3 minutes. Add the turmeric and chicken and stir-fry for 3-4 minutes or until light brown. Season with salt and pepper to taste.

Serving Size 234 g

Amount Per Serving

Calories 209

Calories from Fat 96

Total Fat 10.7g16%

Saturated Fat 2.0g

Cholesterol 38mg

Sodium 197mg

Potassium 625mg

Total Carbohydrates 13.0g

Dietary Fiber 4.2g

Sugars 3.3g

Protein 15.6g

Vitamin A 26% • Vitamin C 58% • Calcium 18%   •   Iron 6%

8. Avocado with strawberry

Fresh fruit, according to the University of Maryland Medical Center, is a food you should eat plenty of while suffering a gallbladder attack. Fruit contains antioxidants, which can help heal your gallbladder. They also contain no cholesterol and little, if any, fat and are easy for your body to digest. When your gallbladder becomes inflamed, irritated or has gallstones, digesting fatty foods and cholesterol becomes extremely challenging. Your gallbladder normally helps your body digest fats and cholesterol, but when it experiences health problems it can't function like it's supposed to until the issues have been resolved.

Ingredients:

1 cup Avocado, stoned, peeled and cut into chunks

1 cup Strawberry, halved

4 Tbsp. Low-fat plain yogurt

1 1/2 cup Almond milk

2 Tbsp. Lemon juice

3/4 cup Honey

Preparation:

Throw in all ingredients in a blender. Blend until consistency is smooth.

Serving Size 249 g

Amount Per Serving

Calories 499

Calories from Fat 260

Total Fat 28.9g

Saturated Fat 20.7g

Trans Fat 0.0g

Cholesterol 1mg

Sodium 31mg

Potassium 547mg

Total Carbohydrates 64.5g

Dietary Fiber 5.3g

Sugars 58.4g

Protein 4.1g

Vitamin A 1% •Vitamin C 52%• Calcium 6% • Iron 12%

9. Garlic and tomato with zucchini pasta

Zucchinis are a good source of vitamin C which transforms cholesterol into bile. It is one of the very low calorie vegetables which contain 17 calories per 100g serving. It contains no saturated fats or cholesterol and its peel contains an adequate amount of fiber. This makes it ideal for weight reduction and may help in gall bladder stone prevention.

Ingredients:

8 oz. Angel hair pasta

2 lbs. Pasta

2 Tbsp. Garlic, crushed

½ cup Zucchini, strips

1 Tbsp. Olive oil

1 tbsp. Basil, chopped

1 Tbsp. Tomato paste

1/8 Salt

1/8 Pepper

Preparation:

Cover tomatoes with water and bring to boil. Stir before it begins to boil. Once it boils, turn off heat and cover.

Cook the pasta in a large pot of boiling salted water until al dente.

In a skillet, over medium heat, sauté garlic and zucchini in olive oil until garlic is opaque and zucchini is tender. Stir in the tomato paste. Immediately stir in the tomatoes. Season with salt and pepper to taste. Reduce heat, and simmer until the pasta is ready. Garnish with fresh basil.

Mix pasta with sauce and transfer to a serving platter.

Serving Size 207 g

Amount Per Serving

Calories 572

Calories from Fat 60

Total Fat 6.7g

Saturated Fat 0.9g

Cholesterol 138mg

Sodium 57mg

Potassium 403mg

Total Carbohydrates 105.2g

Sugars 0.5g

Protein 21.8g

Vitamin A 3% • Vitamin C 5% • Calcium 4% • Iron 36%

10.   Grilled salmon

Research show that consumption of omega 3 fatty acid found in salmon may help prevent gallstones.

Ingredients:

4 to 6 oz. (150 to 200 g) salmon fillets for each serving

Marinade for enough salmon to serve 8:

2 Tbsp. Garlic

1/2 Tsp. Salt

½ tsp. Pepper

¼ cup Fresh lemon juice

1 Tbsp. Thyme

1/2 cup Honey

1/2 cup Water

1/4 cup Olive oil

Preparation:

In a small bowl, combine the garlic, salt, pepper, fresh lemon juice, thyme, honey, water and olive oil. Pour marinade into a large Ziploc plastic bag and place fish inside. Refrigerate for at least 2 hours. Fire up the grill. Lightly brush the grill grate with olive oil. Place the salmon on the grill. After 7 minutes, flip the salmon and cook for another 7 minutes. Transfer to a serving dish with your favorite side dish and enjoy!

Serving Size 270 g

Amount Per Serving

Calories 574

Calories from Fat 262

Total Fat 29.1g

Saturated Fat 4.4g

Trans Fat 0.0g

Cholesterol 25mg

Sodium 620mg

Potassium 352mg

Total Carbohydrates 74.5g

Dietary Fiber 1.1g

Sugars 70.3g

Protein 12.2g

Vitamin A 2% • Vitamin C 30% • Calcium 7% • Iron 15%

11.   Chicken with horseradish salad

Horseradish is known to naturally remove gall stones and its sediment. It is also used to treat urinary tract infection and kidney stones.

Ingredients:

1 cup Cooked chicken, shredded

1 Onion, thinly sliced

1 pack Mesclun greens

1 Tbsp. Olive oil

2 Tbsp. Horseradish, grated

2 Tbsp. Sour cream

2 Tbsp. Light mayonnaise

½ cup Green onions, minced

1 tsp. Apple cider vinegar

1/8 tsp. Salt

1/8 tsp. Pepper

Preparation:

To make the salad dressing, combine olive oil, horseradish, sour cream, green onions, apple cider vinegar, salt, and pepper in a bowl.

In a salad bowl, arrange the onions on top of the mesclun greens. Drizzle with salad dressing and serve.

Serving Size 202 g

Amount Per Serving

Calories 287

Calories from Fat 151

Total Fat 16.8g

Saturated Fat 3.9g

Trans Fat 0.0g

Cholesterol 63mg

Sodium 356mg

Potassium 339mg

Total Carbohydrates 12.8g

Dietary Fiber 2.4g

Sugars 5.1g

Protein 22.1g

Vitamin A 7%•Vitamin C 21% • Calcium 6% • Iron 7%

12.   Strawberry lemon sorbet

Consumption of fruits and vegetables which contain high amounts of water-soluble fiber helps by flushing out toxins from the body. Strawberry and lemon are enriched with vitamin C and antioxidants that may help prevent gallstones formation.

Ingredients:

3 cups Strawberries

1 cup Honey

½ cup Water

1 cup Fresh lemon juice

3 Tbsp. Lemon zest, finely grated

1/8 tsp. Salt

Preparation:

Blend strawberries, lemon juice and lemon zest using a food processor. Add honey one at a time. Then add salt. Refrigerate until well chilled. Pour mixture into an ice cream maker. Scoop into an air tight container. Store in the freezer until ready to serve.

Serving Size 294 g

Amount Per Serving

Calories 310

Calories from Fat 8

Total Fat 0.8g1%

Cholesterol 0mg0%

Sodium 91mg4%

Potassium 299mg9%

Total Carbohydrates 80.3g27%

Dietary Fiber 2.9g11%

Sugars 76.4g

Protein 1.6g

Vitamin A 1% • Vitamin C 162% • Calcium 3% • Iron 5%

Protein 4.0g

Vitamin A 8% • Vitamin C 7% • Calcium 3% • Iron 12%

13.   Chicken with barbecue and applesauce

Studies show that the pectin in apples stops gallstone formation and dissolves stones as well.

Ingredients:

4 Chicken breast fillet

½ tsp. Pepper

1 Tbsp. Olive oil.

2/3 cup Apple sauce

2/3 cup Barbecue sauce

2 Tbsp. Honey

Preparation:

Rub chicken with pepper. In a skillet, over medium heat, brown the chicken in olive oil until both sides are light brown. In a small bowl, combine all remaining ingredients. Pour over chicken. Cover with a lid and continue cooking for another 8 minutes or until meat is thoroughly cooked. Transfer to serving plate and enjoy!

Serving Size 149 g

Amount Per Serving

Calories 267

Calories from Fat 65

Total Fat 7.3g

Saturated Fat 1.0g

Trans Fat 0.0g

Cholesterol 0mg

Sodium 934mg

Potassium 214mg

Total Carbohydrates 51.9g

Dietary Fiber 1.0g

Sugars 42.6g

Protein 0.1g

Vitamin A 4% • Vitamin C 2% • Calcium 1% • Iron 2%

14.   Grilled chicken with thyme

Apple cider vinegar stops the liver from making cholesterol because of its acidic nature. It is used to dissolve gallstones and alleviates the pain caused by the pressing stones.

Ingredients:

350 g. Chicken breasts fillet, butterfly-cut

1 cup Apple Cider Vinegar

3 Tbsp. Thyme

1 Tbsp. Sea Salt

1 Tbsp. Pepper

Preparation:

In a container with lid, combine the apple cider vinegar, thyme, sea salt and pepper. Stir well. Place the chicken in a container, mix thoroughly. Seal with a lid and refrigerate for 20 minutes. Place chicken on warmed grill. Rotate the chicken every 5 minutes. Chicken is finished when juices run clear.

Serving Size 206 g

Amount Per Serving

Calories 225

Calories from Fat 72

Total Fat 8.0g

Saturated Fat 2.2g

Trans Fat 0.0g

Cholesterol 88mg

Sodium 1966mg

Potassium 403mg

Total Carbohydrates 3.8g

Dietary Fiber 1.6g

Protein 29.7g

Vitamin A 3% • Vitamin C 3% • Calcium 23% • Iron 24%

15.   Garlic pasta

Garlic lowers the concentration of cholesterol in bile preventing gallstones formation. It is also used for liver detoxification because of the sulfur that it contains.

Ingredients:

200 g. Vegetable pasta

3/4 cup Extra virgin oil

3/4 cup Garlic, crushed

3/4 cup Parsley

1 cup Button mushroom, halved

Preparation:

Cook the pasta according to its package instruction.

In a skillet, heat the extra virgin oil over medium heat. Add the garlic and sauté until light brown. Add the parsley and mushroom. Lower the heat and simmer for two minutes while stirring. Add the cooked pasta in the skillet.

Serving Size 109 g

Amount Per Serving

Calories 92

Calories from Fat 5

Total Fat 0.5g

Cholesterol 0mg

Sodium 23mg

Potassium 440mg

Total Carbohydrates 19.4g

Dietary Fiber 2.2g

Sugars 1.3g

Protein 5.0g

Vitamin A 38%•Vitamin C 78% • Calcium 12% • Iron 18%

16.   Onion pickled shrimp salad

Onions are a good source of vitamin C because of the phytochemicals it contains. It is a good source of dietary fiber. Studies show that onion reduces the incidence of cholesterol gallstones and helps shrink existing gallstones by reducing the concentration of cholesterol in bile.

Ingredients:

1 Red onion, thinly sliced

1/2 cup Apple cider vinegar

1/2 cup Honey

1/8 tsp. Salt

1/8 tsp. Pepper

300g. Shrimp, steamed

1 bag loosely packed Mesclun greens

Preparation:

To make the salad dressing, in a bowl, combine the red onion, apple cider vinegar, honey, salt and pepper.

Arrange the mesclun greens and the shrimp in a salad bowl. Drizzle the salad dressing on top and enjoy!

Serving Size 234 g

Amount Per Serving

Calories 314

Calories from Fat 16

Total Fat 1.7g

Saturated Fat 0.5g

Trans Fat 0.0g

Cholesterol 211mg

Sodium 347mg

Potassium 283mg

Total Carbohydrates 51.9g

Dietary Fiber 0.9g

Sugars 48.1g

Protein 23.4g

Vitamin A 6% • Vitamin C 5% • Calcium 11% • Iron 4%

17.   Artichoke and shallots

Artichokes are known to prevent gallstones by increasing cynarin, a substance that increases bile production which in turn dissolves cholesterol within the bile.

Ingredients:

9 oz. Frozen artichoke, defrosted and drained

1 cup Shallots

250 g. Chicken breast fillet

3 Tbsp. Olive oil

1/8 tsp. Pepper

4 Tbsp. Olive oil

1 tsp. Lemon juice

Preparation:

In a skillet, over medium-heat, add the olive oil and sauté the shallots until tender. Add the chicken and cook thoroughly for about 5 minutes per side or until light brown. Add the artichoke and bay leaves. Stir for a minute, add the lemon juice and season with salt and pepper.

Serving Size 258 g

Amount Per Serving

Calories 517

Calories from Fat 351

Total Fat 39.0g

Saturated Fat 6.4g

Cholesterol 74mg

Sodium 158mg

Potassium 699mg

Total Carbohydrates 18.0g

Dietary Fiber 4.6g

Sugars 0.9g

Protein 28.2g

Vitamin A 14% • Vitamin C 25% • Calcium 7% • Iron 15%

18.   Blackberry cobbler

Blackberries are rich in water soluble fiber that aids in digestion and lowers cholesterol levels which may help prevent gallstones formation.

Ingredients:

½ cup Olive oil

1 cup Honey

1 cup Flour

1 cup Almond milk

2 cups Fresh blackberries

Preparation:

Preheat the oven to 350F. Grease a baking dish with olive oil.

Using a blender, mix flour, honey, olive oil and milk until well-combined. Pour mixture into a baking dish. Add the blackberries on top of the batter.

Bake the cobbler for one hour or until batter turns golden brown. Cool and serve.

Serving Size 157 g

Amount Per Serving

Calories 432

Calories from Fat 207

Total Fat 22.9g

Saturated Fat 9.3g

Cholesterol 0mg

Sodium 8mg

Potassium 201mg

Total Carbohydrates 59.4g

Dietary Fiber 3.5g

Sugars 43.0g

Protein 3.4g

Vitamin A 2% • Vitamin C 16% • Calcium 2% • Iron 10%

19.　　Cold creamy papaya soup

Papaya is known to improve digestion because of its high water, enzyme and soluble fiber content. Its roots in particular are beneficial in treating gall bladder stones.

Ingredients:

1 Ripe papaya, cut into chunks

2 Tbsp. Lime juice, fresh

1 Tbsp. Honey

1 cup Apple juice

Preparation:

In a food processor, puree the papaya until smooth. Pour into a bowl. Stir in honey, lime juice, and apple juice. Refrigerate. Serve chilled.

Serving Size 425 g

Amount Per Serving

Calories 311

Calories from Fat 11

Total Fat 1.2g

Cholesterol 0mg

Sodium 37mg

Potassium 834mg

Total Carbohydrates 79.4g

Dietary Fiber 6.0g

Sugars 65.8g

Protein 1.8g

Vitamin A 61% • Vitamin C 322% • Calcium 9% • Iron 6%

20.   Mango pear smoothie

One mango contains half of the recommended daily allowance of vitamin C, essential in preventing gallstones formation. Pears contain pectin which binds to the cholesterol-filled gallstones helping it flush out easily.

Ingredients:

3 Pears, cored

2 cups Mangoes, cubed

Preparation:

In a blender, combine pears and mangoes. Blend well, transfer to chilled glasses and enjoy!

Serving Size 276 g

Amount Per Serving

Calories 255

Calories from Fat 10

Total Fat 1.2g

Cholesterol 0mg

Sodium 5mg

Potassium 618mg

Total Carbohydrates 65.2g

Dietary Fiber 9.8g

Sugars 51.0g

Protein 2.6g

Vitamin A 22%• Vitamin C 79% • Calcium 3% • Iron 3%

21.   Flax with fresh lemon juice vinegar

Flax seed and lemon juice are a winning combination for treating gallstones. The soluble fiber content of flax seed traps cholesterol and fat making it not absorbable by the body. The lignans in flaxseed contain high amount of fiber and is enriched with an antioxidant property. The pectin in lemon helps flush out gallstones.

Ingredients:

½ cup Cucumber, chopped

1 cup Apple, cored and sliced

½ cup Strawberries

1 cup Spinach

1/2 cup Lemon juice

2 Tbsp. Honey

1 Tbsp. Flax seed, freshly grinded

1 cup water

Ice

Preparation:

Combine everything and blend until smooth. Enjoy!

Serving Size 213 g

Amount Per Serving

Calories 174

Calories from Fat 18

Total Fat 2.0g

Saturated Fat 0.7g

Trans Fat 0.0g

Cholesterol 0mg

Sodium 28mg

Potassium 411mg

Total Carbohydrates 39.2g

Dietary Fiber 5.1g

Sugars 32.4g

Protein 2.3g

Vitamin A 29% • Vitamin C 105% • Calcium 3% • Iron 12%

22.   Baked potatoes with hemp dressing

Including omega 3 fatty acid in one's diet is beneficial in maintaining a healthy bladder and in preventing gallstone formation.

Ingredients:

2 Potatoes, scrubbed and rinsed

1 cup Water

2 Tbsp. Low-fat plain yogurt

1 cup Shelled hemp seeds

½ Tbsp. Onion, minced

½ Tbsp. Garlic, minced

1 Tbsp. Apple cider vinegar

1 Tbsp. Fresh dill

2 Tbsp. Chives

1/8 tsp. salt

Preparation:

Pierce the potatoes using the tines of the fork. Bake potatoes in 425F for 45 to 60 minutes using a conventional oven toaster.

To make the dressing combine all remaining ingredients except dill and chives in a food processor and blend well.

Drizzle on top of baked potatoes. Garnish with dill and chives. Transfer to a serving platter and enjoy.

Serving Size 364 g

Amount Per Serving

Calories 168

Calories from Fat 5

Total Fat 0.5g

Trans Fat 0.0g

Cholesterol 1mg

Sodium 178mg

Potassium 982mg

Total Carbohydrates 36.5g

Dietary Fiber 5.5g

Sugars 3.8g

Protein 5.0g

Vitamin A 5% • Vitamin C 76% • Calcium 9% • Iron 11%

23.   Cucumber and beet salad

Beets contain anti-inflammatory, antioxidant and detoxifying properties beneficial for gallstones prevention. It promotes healthy bile flow. Cucumber provides hydration and fiber that help prevent gallstones formation.

Ingredients:

4 beets, thinly sliced

¾ cup Cucumber, thinly sliced

6 scallions, cut into 2"

Zest of 1 lemon, grated

5 oz. Low-fat cottage cheese, grated

1 cup Parsley

¼ cup Apple cider vinegar

1 Tbsp. Honey

1 tsp. Poppy seeds

Kosher salt, freshly ground pepper

Olive oil (for drizzling)

Preparation:

In a large bowl, toss in beets, cucumbers, scallions, lemon

zest, cheese and parsley. Add apple cider vinegar, honey and poppy seeds. Season with salt and pepper. Drizzle with olive oil. Mix salad and enjoy!

Serving Size 214 g

Amount Per Serving

Calories 116

Calories from Fat 14

Total Fat 1.5g

Saturated Fat 0.6g

Trans Fat 0.0g

Cholesterol 3mg

Sodium 273mg

Potassium 531mg

Total Carbohydrates 19.2g

Dietary Fiber 3.3g

Sugars 13.5g

Protein 7.7g

Vitamin A 31% • Vitamin C 47% • Calcium 9% • Iron 13

24.   Watercress and celery smoothie

Watercress is rich in vitamin C. Native Indians reportedly used watercress to dissolve gallstones.

Ingredients:

1 cup tightly packed Watercress

1 cup Celery chunks

1 cup Almond milk

1 Tbsp. Honey

2 Ice cubes

Preparation:

Combine all ingredients and blend well. Enjoy chilled!

Serving Size 131 g

Amount Per Serving

Calories 308

Calories from Fat 257

Total Fat 28.6g

Saturated Fat 25.4g

Cholesterol 0mg

Sodium 18mg

Potassium 321mg

Total Carbohydrates 15.3g

Dietary Fiber 2.7g

Sugars 12.6g

Protein 2.8g

Vitamin A 0% • Vitamin C 6% • Calcium 2% •Iron 11%

25. Dandelion orange smoothie

Dandelions are a good source of calcium, iron, vitamins A and C. It stimulates a healthy bile flow effectively promoting blood purity. It is also used to cleanse the liver.

Ingredients:

1 cup Organic dandelion leaves

1 Navel orange, peeled

1 cup Strawberry yogurt

2 Ice cubes

Preparation:

Throw in all ingredients in a blender. Shake well and enjoy!

Serving Size 429 g

Amount Per Serving

Calories 329

Calories from Fat 27

Total Fat 3.0g

Saturated Fat 1.9g

Cholesterol 12mg

Sodium 130mg

Potassium 767mg

Total Carbohydrates 67.3g

Dietary Fiber 4.4g

Sugars 62.9g

Protein 11.5g

Vitamin A 10% • Vitamin C 166% • Calcium 41% • Iron 2%

26.   Beet greens sandwich

Beet greens are rich in calcium, iron, magnesium, vitamin C, manganese, and other vitamins and stimulate healthy bile flow. The betaine in beet greens makes this vegetable excellent for liver detoxification.

Ingredients:

2 slices Whole wheat bread

1 tsp. Garlic, minced

3 oz. Skim ricotta cheese, cubed

1 bunch Beet greens, blanched and chopped

½ tsp. Extra virgin oil

1 cup Beet, sliced into strips

Preparation:

Rub surface of the bread with garlic. Spread ricotta cheese over the bread. Layer with beets, beet greens and cheese alternately. Drizzle with olive oil. Toast in the oven toaster for 3 to 4 minutes or until cheese has melted. Serve and enjoy!

Serving Size 229 g

Amount Per Serving

Calories 297

Calories from Fat 79

Total Fat 8.8g

Saturated Fat 4.6g

Trans Fat 0.5g

Cholesterol 26mg

Sodium 437mg

Potassium 516mg

Total Carbohydrates 36.9g

Dietary Fiber 5.6g

Sugars 10.2g

Protein 18.5g

Vitamin A 7%•Vitamin C 7%•Calcium 31%•Iron 14%

27.   Baby mixed organic greens Italian salad

A diet rich in green vegetables is important in the treatment and prevention of gallstones because of its high dietary fiber content. A diet low in calories is ideal in achieving a healthy body weight essential in managing gallbladder symptoms.

Ingredients:

1 pack Baby mixed organic greens

½ cup Extra virgin olive oil

2 Tbsp. Apple cider vinegar

2 Tbsp. Fresh lemon juice

2 Tbsp. Fresh parsley, chopped

1 Tbsp. Garlic, minced

1 tsp. Fresh oregano, finely chopped

1 tsp. Fresh marjoram, finely chopped

1 Tbsp. Honey

1/8 tsp. Salt

1/8 tsp. Pepper

Preparation:

Whisk in all ingredients in a bowl. Add in the vegetables. Mix then transfer to a serving platter and enjoy!

Serving Size 104 g

Amount Per Serving

Calories 482

Calories from Fat 456

Total Fat 50.7g

Saturated Fat 7.3g

Trans Fat 0.0g

Cholesterol 0mg

Sodium 155mg

Potassium 92mg

Total Carbohydrates 11.5g

Dietary Fiber 0.8g

Sugars 9.1g

Protein 0.7g

Vitamin A 8% • Vitamin C 23% • Calcium 3% •Iron 6%

28. Low-fat strawberry muffin

Strawberries contain a high amount of antioxidants, manganese, dietary fiber and vitamin C all beneficial in managing gallstones.

Ingredients:

1 1/2 cups all-purpose flour

1/2 cup Honey

2 1/2 tsp. Baking powder

1 tsp. Ground cinnamon

1/4 tsp. Salt

2/3 cup Fat-free plain yogurt

1/4 cup Olive oil

3 Tbsp. Skim milk

1 large Egg, lightly beaten

1/4 cup Strawberry jam

½ tsp. Ground cinnamon

Preparation:

Preheat the oven to 375F. Put liners in muffin cups. Grease liners with olive oil using a spray.

In a large bowl, combine flour, honey, baking powder, ground cinnamon and salt. Mix well using a whisk. Make a well in the center of the mixture. Combine yogurt, olive oil, skim milk and egg in a bowl. Stir well. Add yogurt mixture to flour mixture. Stir until moist.

Spoon 1 tablespoon of batter into each liner. Put 1 teaspoon of strawberry jam on top, then cover with the remaining batter. Sprinkle cinnamon over batter. Bake for 15 minutes or until wooden tooth pick inserted in center comes out clean. Cool and serve.

Serving Size 129 g

Amount Per Serving

Calories 409

Calories from Fat 103

Total Fat 11.5g

Saturated Fat 1.8g

Trans Fat 0.0g

Cholesterol 37mg

Sodium 140mg

Potassium 341mg

Total Carbohydrates 73.7g

Dietary Fiber 1.5g

Sugars 28.5g

Protein 5.6g

Vitamin A 1% • Vitamin C 0% • Calcium 14% • Iron 13%

29.   Bladder cleanse smoothie

Oranges contain pectin that provides a high amount of dietary fiber. It also contains vitamin C which may prevent gallstones formation.

Ingredients:

3 Orange navels, chopped

1 cup Fresh grapefruit, chopped

3 Tbsp. Epsom salt

½ cup olive oil.

3 Ice cubes

Preparation:

Combine all ingredients and blend. Serve chilled. Enjoy in the evening before going to bed.

Serving Size 338 g

Amount Per Serving

Calories 938

Calories from Fat 909

Total Fat 101.0g

Saturated Fat 14.4g

Cholesterol 0mg

Sodium 0mg

Potassium 320mg

Total Carbohydrates 18.6g

Dietary Fiber 2.5g

Sugars 16.1g

Protein 1.4g

Vitamin A 43% • Vitamin C 132% • Calcium 3% • Iron 1%

30.   Apple lemon bladder cleanse smoothie

Apple contains pectin that is very high in dietary fiber which helps reduce cholesterol by reducing the amount of it being absorbed in the intestines. It is extremely rich in important antioxidants and flavonoids.

Ingredients:

3 cups Apple, cored and chopped

3/4 cup Juice of fresh lemon

1 cup Low-fat yogurt

½ cup Olive oil

1 Tbsp. Honey

Preparation:

Combine all ingredients and blend well. Transfer to chilled glasses and enjoy!

Serving Size 225 g

Amount Per Serving

Calories 483

Calories from Fat 315

Total Fat 35.0g

Saturated Fat 5.6g

Trans Fat 0.0g

Cholesterol 5mg

Sodium 59mg

Potassium 433mg

Total Carbohydrates 42.3g

Dietary Fiber 5.4g

Sugars 34.7g

Protein 5.3g

Vitamin A 1% • Vitamin C 29% • Calcium 15% • Iron 6%

31.   Strawberry grapefruit shake

Grapefruit is used for gallbladder cleansing because it contains limonoid, a substance that dissolves gallstones. Gallstones also increases calcium excretion and can help prevent gallstone formation in the future.

Ingredients:

1 cup Grapefruit

1 cup Strawberries, chopped

1 cup Low-fat plain yogurt

1 Tbsp. Honey

3 Ice cubes

Preparation:

Combine all ingredients, blend well and enjoy!

Serving Size 320 g

Amount Per Serving

Calories 179

Calories from Fat 17

Total Fat 1.8g

Saturated Fat 1.2g

Cholesterol 7mg

Sodium 87mg

Potassium 562mg

Total Carbohydrates 32.1g

Dietary Fiber 2.7g

Sugars 28.8g

Protein 8.2g

Vitamin A 23% • Vitamin C 138% • Calcium 25% • Iron 3%

32.   Toasted wheat bread with artichoke dip

Artichokes have been used since ancient times as an aid for indigestion. It has a powerful antioxidant and lipid-lowering properties. It also promotes healthy bile flow.

Ingredients:

1 bag (8oz.) Pita chips

2 Tbsp. Garlic, minced

2 Tbsp. Green onions, minced

1 cup Avocado, mashed

2 Tbsp. Fat-free cream cheese

1/2 cup Ricotta cheese, grated

1 can (14 oz.) Artichoke hearts, chopped in chunks

1 pack (10 oz.) Spinach, finely chopped

1/8 Salt

1/8 Pepper

½ Tbsp. Olive oil

Preparation:

Preheat the oven to 350F.

Grease an oven-safe dish with olive oil.

Combine avocado, cream cheese, and ricotta cheese. Mix well. Add all remaining ingredients except the pita chips. Transfer avocado with artichokes mixture to the oven-safe dish. Cook the dish for 30 minutes or until top is golden brown.

Serve with pita chips and enjoy!

Serving Size 305 g

Amount Per Serving

Calories 347

Calories from Fat 241

Total Fat 26.7g

Saturated Fat 8.8g

Trans Fat 0.0g

Cholesterol 30mg

Sodium 238mg

Potassium 1286mg

Total Carbohydrates 18.1g

Dietary Fiber 8.3g

Sugars 1.4g

Protein 13.9g

Vitamin A 277% • Vitamin C 85% • Calcium 35% • Iron 27%

33.   Parsley pesto sandwich

Almonds are a good source of magnesium and calcium which help prevent gallstones formation by binding bile acids in the intestines. It also aids in lowering cholesterol levels and have excellent antioxidant effects.

Ingredients:

2 slices Whole wheat bread

1/2 cup Almonds, blanched

1 cup Fresh parsley

2 Tbsp. Garlic

1/8 tsp. Salt

1/2 cup Ricotta cheese, grated

1 cup Olive oil

Preparation:

Throw in all ingredients in a food processor and blend well.

Spread on sandwich slices and enjoy!

Serving Size 211 g

Amount Per Serving

Calories 878

Calories from Fat 724

Total Fat 80.5g

Saturated Fat 12.7g

Trans Fat 0.5g

Cholesterol 13mg

Sodium 425mg

Potassium 440mg

Total Carbohydrates 31.8g

Dietary Fiber 6.6g26%

Sugars 4.1g

Protein 16.3g

Vitamin A 37% • Vitamin C 47% • Calcium 25% • Iron 19%

34.　　Guava spread

Guavas are a good source of vitamins A and C. Vitamin C is vital for converting cholesterol into bile acids. One guava fruit contains 4 times more vitamin C than an average-size orange.

Ingredients:

8 cups Ripe guava, washed, peeled, chopped in chunks and mashed

1 packet MCP pectin powder

4 cups Honey

 1/4 cup Lemon juice

½ tsp. Olive oil

Preparation:

In a large saucepan, over low-medium heat place the guavas, then add the honey, lemon juice and olive oil. Gently stir in the ingredients. Boil the mixture and stir constantly to avoid burning the fruit. Let the fruit mixture simmer for 5-20 minutes until it reaches a thick consistency similar to syrup. Remove from heat. Remove any foam or bubbles on top of the surface. Store in a well-cleaned and sealed jar then cool and refrigerate. Once cooled, scoop a spoonful of jam and spread on the sandwich. Enjoy!

Serving Size 274 g

Amount Per Serving

Calories 505

Calories from Fat 14

Total Fat 1.5g

Cholesterol 0mg

Sodium 9mg

Potassium 629mg

Total Carbohydrates 130.8g

Dietary Fiber 7.4g

Sugars 123.2g

Protein 3.8g

Vitamin A 16% • Vitamin C 508% • Calcium 3% • Iron 5%

JUICES

1.   Fennel Collard Greens Juice

Ingredients:

1 large fennel bulb

1 cup of collard greens

1 large leek

1 cup of mustard greens

1 medium-sized Granny Smith apple, cored

1 large cucumber

Preparation:

Wash the fennel bulb and trim off the wilted outer layers. Cut into small chunks and set aside.

Combine collard greens and mustard greens in a large pot. Add 2 cups of hot water and soak for 15 minutes. Drain and set aside.

Wash the leek and roughly chop it. Set aside.

Wash the cucumber and cut into thick slices. Set aside.

Wash the apple and remove the core. Cut into bite-sized pieces and set aside.

Now, process fennel, collard greens, mustard greens, leek, cucumber, and apple in a juicer.

Transfer to serving glasses and add some ice before serving.

Enjoy!

Nutritional information per serving: Kcal: 223, Protein: 9.6g, Carbs: 67.9g, Fats: 1.8g

2.   Celery Sweet Potato Juice

Ingredients:

1 cup of celery, chopped

1 cup of sweet potato, chopped

1 cup of Swiss chard, torn

1 large cucumber

A handful of spinach, torn

2 oz of water

Preparation:

Wash the celery and chop into small pieces. Set aside.

Peel the sweet potato and cut into chunks. Fill the measuring cup and reserve the rest for some other juice.

Combine Swiss chard and spinach in a colander. Wash thoroughly under cold running water and torn with hands. Drain and set aside.

Wash the cucumber and cut into thick slices. Set aside.

Now, combine celery, sweet potato, Swiss chard, cucumber, and spinach in a juicer and process until juiced. Transfer to serving glasses and stir in the water.

Refrigerate for 10 minutes before serving.

Enjoy!

Nutritional information per serving: Kcal: 156, Protein: 6.3g, Carbs: 43.2g, Fats: 0.8g

3.   Artichoke Spring Onion Juice

Ingredients:

1 large artichoke

½ cup of spring onions, roughly chopped

1 cup of asparagus, trimmed

1 large cucumber

1 small green apple, cored

1 small ginger root knob, 1-inch

Preparation:

Using a sharp knife, trim off the outer leaves of the artichoke. Wash it and cut into small pieces. Set aside.

Place the spring onions in a colander and wash under cold running water. Drain and roughly chop. Set aside.

Wash the asparagus and trim off the woody ends. Chop into small pieces and set aside.

Wash the cucumber and cut into thick slices. Set aside.

Wash the apple and remove the core. Cut into bite-sized pieces and set aside.

Peel the ginger root knob and set aside.

Now, process artichoke, spring onions, asparagus, cucumber, apple, and ginger root in a juicer.

Transfer to serving glasses and add some ice.

Serve immediately.

Nutritional information per serving: Kcal: 181, Protein: 11.4g, Carbs: 57.5g, Fats: 1.1g

4.   Fuji Banana Juice

Ingredients:

1 large Fuji apple, cored

1 large orange

1 large banana

1 medium-sized zucchini

2 oz of water

Preparation:

Wash the apple and remove the core. Cut into bite-sized pieces and set aside.

Peel the orange and divide into wedges. Set aside.

Peel the banana and cut into small chunks. Set aside.

Peel the zucchini and cut in half. Scoop out the seeds and cut into small pieces. Set aside.

Now, process apple, orange, banana, and zucchini in a juicer.

Transfer to serving glasses and refrigerate for 15 minutes before serving.

Enjoy!

Nutritional information per serving: Kcal: 296, Protein: 6.5g, Carbs: 86.8g, Fats: 1.7g

5.   Golden Pineapple Juice

Ingredients:

1 cup of pineapple chunks

1 large orange

1 large lemon

1 small Golden Delicious apple, cored

1 cup of celery, chopped

2 oz of water

1 tbsp of honey

Preparation:

Cut the top of a pineapple and peel it using a sharp knife. Cut into small chunks. Reserve the rest of the pineapple in a refrigerator for some other juice.

Peel the orange and divide into wedges. Set aside.

Peel the lemon and cut lengthwise in half. Set aside.

Wash the apple and remove the core. Cut into bite-sized pieces and set aside.

Wash the celery and chop into small pieces. Set aside.

Now, combine pineapple, orange, lemon, apple, and celery in a juicer and process until juiced.

Transfer to serving glasses and stir in the water and honey. Add some ice and serve immediately.

Enjoy!

Nutritional information per serving: Kcal: 284, Protein: 4.3g, Carbs: 69.2g, Fats: 0.9g

6. Cherry Cantaloupe Juice

Ingredients:

1 cup of cherries

1 large green apple, cored

1 cup of cantaloupe, chopped

1 large carrot

2 oz of water

Preparation:

Place the cherries in a colander and wash under cold running water. Drain and cut in half. Remove the pits and set aside.

Wash the apple and remove the core. Cut into bite-sized pieces and set aside.

Cut the cantaloupe in half. Scoop out the seeds and cut two large wedges. Peel and chop into chunks. Reserve the rest of the cantaloupe in a refrigerator for some other juice.

Wash the carrot and cut into thick slices. Set aside.

Now, combine cherries, apple, cantaloupe, and carrot in a juicer and process until juiced.

Transfer to serving glasses and stir in the water. Add some ice or refrigerate before serving.

Nutritional information per serving: Kcal: 249, Protein: 4.5g, Carbs: 72.3g, Fats: 1.1g

7.   Papaya Blueberry Juice

Ingredients:

1 small papaya

1 cup of blueberries

1 medium-sized orange

1 cup of watermelon

1 large cucumber

2 oz of water

1 tbsp agave nectar

Preparation:

Peel the papaya and cut lengthwise in half. Scoop out the black seeds and flesh using a spoon. Cut into small chunks and set aside.

Wash the blueberries under cold running water. Drain and set aside.

Peel the orange and divide into wedges. Set aside.

Cut the watermelon lengthwise. For one cup, you will need about one large wedge. Peel and cut into chunks. Remove the seeds and set aside. Reserve the rest of the melon for some other juices.

Wash the cucumber and cut into thick slices. Set aside.

Now, process papaya, blueberries, orange, watermelon, and cucumber in a juicer. Transfer to serving glasses and stir in the water and agave nectar.

Add some ice and serve immediately.

Nutritional information per serving: Kcal: 320, Protein: 6g, Carbs: 76.2g, Fats: 1.6g

8.   Zucchini Broccoli Juice

Ingredients:

1 large zucchini

1 cup of broccoli, chopped

3 large leeks, chopped

1 cup of fresh parsley, torn

A handful of spinach, torn

2 oz of water

Preparation:

Peel the zucchini and cut in half. Scoop out the seeds and chop into small pieces. Set aside.

Wash the broccoli and chop into small pieces. Set aside.

Wash the leeks and roughly chop them. Set aside.

Wash the parsley and spinach thoroughly and torn with hands. Set aside.

Now, combine zucchini, broccoli, leeks, parsley, and spinach in a juicer and process until juiced.

Transfer to serving glasses and stir in the water. Add some ice and serve immediately.

Enjoy!

Nutritional information per serving: Kcal: 225, Protein: 13.1g, Carbs: 58.7g, Fats: 2.7g

9.   Strawberry Cranberry Juice

Ingredients:

1 cup of strawberries

1 large Fuji apple, cored

1 cup of cranberries

1 large carrot

1 large lemon

1 large orange

Preparation:

Place the strawberries and cranberries in a colander and wash under cold running water. Drain and cut in half. Set aside.

Wash the apple and remove the core. Cut into bite-sized pieces and set aside.

Wash the carrot and cut into thick slices. Set aside.

Peel the lemon cut lengthwise in half. Set aside.

Peel the orange and divide into wedges. Set aside.

Now, process strawberries, apple, cranberries, carrots, lemon, and orange in juicer. Transfer to serving glasses and stir in the water.

Add few ice cubes, or refrigerate for 15 minutes before serving.

Nutritional information per serving: Kcal: 268, Protein: 5.6g, Carbs: 89.1g, Fats: 1.6g

10. Beet Lime Juice

Ingredients:

3 large beets, trimmed

1 large lime

1 large cucumber

2 celery stalk, chopped

1 small ginger root knob, 1-inch

2 oz of water

Preparation:

Wash the beets and trim off the green parts. Cut into small pieces and set aside.

Peel the lime and cut lengthwise in half. Set aside.

Wash the cucumber and cut into thick slices. Set aside.

Wash the celery and chop into bite-sized pieces. Set aside.

Peel the ginger root knob and set aside.

Now, combine beets, lime, cucumber, celery, and ginger in a juicer and process until juiced. Transfer to serving glasses and stir in the water.

Refrigerate for 20 minutes before serving.

Nutritional information per serving: Kcal: 140, Protein: 6.7g, Carbs: 41.6g, Fats: 0.9g

11. Coconut Blackberry Juice

Ingredients:

1 cup of blackberries

1 large orange

1 large yellow apple

1 cup of fresh mint, torn

1 tbsp honey

3 oz coconut water

Preparation:

Place the blackberries in a colander and wash under cold running water. Drain and set aside.

Peel the orange and divide into wedges. Set aside.

Wash the apple and remove the core. Cut into bite-sized pieces and set aside.

Place the mint in a bowl and add one cup of lukewarm water. Let it soak for 15 minutes.

Now, combine blackberries, orange, apple, and mint in a juicer and process until juiced.

Transfer to serving glasses and stir in the coconut water and honey. Add some ice and serve immediately.

Enjoy!

Nutritional information per serving: Kcal: 287, Protein: 5.3g, Carbs: 88.4g, Fats: 1.5g

12. Avocado Pomegranate Juice

Ingredients:

1 cup of avocado

1 cup of pomegranate seeds

1 large cucumber

1 large carrot

¼ tsp of nutmeg

3 oz of water

Preparation:

Peel the avocado and cut in half. Remove the pit and cut into small chunks. Set aside.

Cut the top of the pomegranate fruit using a sharp knife. Slice down to each of the white membranes inside of the fruit. Pop the seeds into a bowl and set aside.

Wash the cucumber and carrot. Cut into thick slices and set aside.

Now, combine avocado, pomegranate seeds, cucumber, and carrot in a juicer and process until juiced.

Transfer to serving glasses and stir in the water and nutmeg. Add some ice and serve immediately.

Enjoy!

Nutritional information per serving: Kcal: 319, Protein: 7.1g, Carbs: 46.9g, Fats: 23.5g

13.   Sweet Potato Tomato Juice

Ingredients:

1 cup of sweet potatoes, cubed

2 large Roma tomatoes

1 cup of Swiss chard, torn

1 cup of fresh basil, torn

1 cup of beet greens, torn

¼ tsp of Himalayan salt

2 oz of water

Preparation:

Wash the tomatoes and place them in a bowl. Cut into small pieces and reserve the juice while cutting. Set aside.

Peel the sweet potato and cut into cubes. Fill the measuring cup and reserve the rest for some other juice. Set aside.

Combine Swiss chard, basil, and beet greens in a colander and wash under cold running water. Drain and set aside.

Now, process tomatoes, sweet potato, and Swiss chard, basil, and beet greens in a juicer.

Transfer to serving glasses and stir in the salt and water.

Refrigerate for 20 minutes before serving.

Nutritional information per serving: Kcal: 157, Protein: 7.5g, Carbs: 44.5g, Fats: 1.1g

14.   Cantaloupe Squash Juice

Ingredients:

1 cup of cantaloupe, chopped

1 cup of butternut squash, chopped

2 large carrots

1 large cucumber

¼ tsp of turmeric, ground

2 oz of water

Preparation:

Cut the cantaloupe in half. Scoop out the seeds and flesh. Cut two medium wedges and peel them. Chop into chunks and set aside. Reserve the rest of the cantaloupe in a refrigerator for some other juice.

Peel the butternut squash and remove the seeds using a spoon. Cut into small cubes and reserve the rest of the squash for some other recipe. Wrap in a plastic foil and refrigerate.

Wash the carrots and cucumber and cut into thick slices. Set aside.

Now, combine cantaloupe, butternut squash, carrots, and cucumber in a juicer and process until juiced.

Transfer to serving glasses and stir in the turmeric and water.

Refrigerate for 10 minutes before serving.

Enjoy!

Nutritional information per serving: Kcal: 182, Protein: 6g, Carbs: 53.8g, Fats: 1.1g

15.   Pineapple Plum Juice

Ingredients:

1 cup of pineapple chunks

3 large plums, pitted

1 cup of watermelon, chopped

1 large Granny Smith apple, cored

2 oz of coconut water

Preparation:

Cut the top of a pineapple and peel it using a sharp knife. Cut into small chunks. Reserve the rest of the pineapple in a refrigerator.

Wash the plums and cut in half. Remove the pits and set aside.

Cut the watermelon lengthwise. For one cup, you will need about one large wedge. Peel and cut into chunks. Remove the seeds and set aside. Reserve the rest of the melon for some other juices.

Wash the apple and remove the core. Cut into bite-sized pieces and set aside.

Now, combine pineapple, plums, watermelon, and apple in a juicer and process until juiced.

Transfer to serving glasses and stir in the coconut water.

Add some ice cubes and serve immediately.

Enjoy!

Nutritional information per serving: Kcal: 301, Protein: 4.1g, Carbs: 83.7g, Fats: 1.3g

16.   Grape Melon Juice

Ingredients:

1 cup of green grapes

1 cup of red grapes

1 large Honeydew melon wedge

1 large banana

2 oz of water

Preparation:

Combine green and red grapes in a colander and wash under cold running water. Drain and set aside.

Cut the honeydew melon lengthwise in half. Scoop out the seeds using a spoon. Cut one large wedge and peel it. Cut into small chunks and place in a bowl. Wrap the rest of the melon in a plastic foil and refrigerate.

Peel the banana and cut into small chunks. Set aside.

Now, combine grapes, honeydew melon, and banana in a juicer.

Transfer to serving glasses and stir in the water. Add some ice before serving.

Enjoy!

Nutritional information per serving: Kcal: 374, Protein: 4.4g, Carbs: 105g, Fats: 1.7g

17.   Apple Mint Juice

Ingredients:

1 large red apple, cored

1 large carrot

1 large cucumber

1 large orange

1 cup of fresh mint

Preparation:

Wash the apple and remove the core. Cut into bite-sized pieces and set aside.

Wash the carrot and cucumber. Cut into thick slices and set aside.

Peel the orange and divide into wedges. Set aside.

Wash the mint and drain. Place it in a bowl and add 1 cup of hot water. Let it soak for 10 minutes. Drain again and set aside.

Now, combine apple, carrots, cucumber, orange, and mint in a juicer and process until juiced. Transfer to serving glasses and add some ice cubes.

Serve immediately.

Nutritional information per serving: Kcal: 268, Protein: 6g, Carbs: 79.7g, Fats: 1.5g

18.   Cherry Cauliflower Juice

Ingredients:

1 cup of cherries

1 small cauliflower head

1 large orange

1 large carrot

1 tbsp of honey

2 oz of water

Preparation:

Wash the cherries under cold running water. Drain and cut in half. Remove the pits and set aside.

Trim off the outer leaves of cauliflower. Wash it and cut into small pieces. Set aside.

Peel the orange and divide into wedges. Set aside.

Wash the carrot and cut into thick slices. Set aside.

Now, process cherries, cauliflower, orange, and carrot in a juicer. Transfer to serving glasses and stir in the honey and water.

Add few ice cubes or refrigerate for 10 minutes before serving.

Enjoy!

Nutritional information per serving: Kcal: 219, Protein: 9.1g, Carbs: 66.3g, Fats: 1.4g

19. Strawberry Cranberry Juice

Ingredients:

1 cup of strawberries, chopped

1 cup of cranberries

1 large green apple, cored

1 cup of fresh kale

1 large cucumber

Preparation:

Combine strawberries and cranberries in a colander and wash under cold running water. Drain and cut strawberries in half. Set aside.

Wash the apple and remove the core. Cut into bite-sized pieces and set aside.

Wash the kale thoroughly and drain. Torn with hands and set aside.

Wash the cucumber and cut into thick slices. Set aside.

Now, process strawberries, cranberries, apple, kale, and cucumber. Transfer to serving glasses and add some ice cubes before serving.

Enjoy!

Nutritional information per serving: Kcal: 229, Protein: 7.4g, Carbs: 72g, Fats: 1.9g

20.   Mango Grapefruit Juice

Ingredients:

1 cup of mango chunks

1 large carrot

1 large grapefruit

1 large lemon

1 small pear, cored

2 oz of water

Preparation:

Wash the mango and cut into chunks. Fill the measuring cup and reserve the rest for some other juice. Set aside.

Wash the carrot and cut into thick slices. Set aside.

Peel the grapefruit and divide into wedges. Set aside.

Peel the lemon and cut lengthwise in half. Set aside.

Wash the pear and remove the core. Cut into bite-sized pieces and set aside.

Now, process mango, carrot, grapefruit, lemon, and pear in a juicer.

Transfer to serving glasses and add stir in the water. Add some ice cubes or refrigerate for 10 minutes before serving.

Enjoy!

Nutritional information per serving: Kcal: 297, Protein: 5.7g, Carbs: 92.7g, Fats: 1.7g

21.   Kiwi Avocado Juice

Ingredients:

3 large kiwis, peeled

1 cup of avocado chunks

1 large cucumber

1 cup of fresh mint

¼ tsp of vanilla extract

3 oz of water

Preparation:

Peel the kiwis and cut lengthwise in half. Set aside.

Peel the avocado and cut in half. Remove the pit and cut into chunks. Reserve the rest for some other juice. Set aside.

Wash the cucumber and cut into thick slices. Set aside.

Wash the mint thoroughly under cold running water. Set aside.

Now, combine kiwis, avocado, cucumber, and mint in a juicer and process until juiced. Transfer to serving glasses and stir in the water and vanilla extract.

Add some ice and serve immediately.

Enjoy!

Nutritional information per serving: Kcal: 351, Protein: 8.3g, Carbs: 57.8g, Fats: 23.6g

22.   Artichoke Pea Juice

Ingredients:

1 large artichoke

1 cup of green peas

1 cup of collard greens, torn

1 medium-sized apple, cored

1 cup of carrots, sliced

¼ tsp of Himalayan salt

2 oz of water

Preparation:

Using a sharp knife, trim off the outer layers of the artichoke. Wash it and cut into bite-sized pieces. Set aside.

Place the green peas in a colander and wash under cold running water. Drain and set aside.

Wash the collard greens thoroughly and torn with hands. Set aside.

Wash the carrots and slice into thin slices. Fill the measuring cup and reserve the rest for some other juice. Set aside.

Now, process artichoke, green peas, collard greens, and carrots in a juicer. Transfer to serving glasses and refrigerate for 10 minutes before serving.

Nutritional information per serving: Kcal: 250, Protein: 16.2g, Carbs: 74.9g, Fats: 1.7g

23.   Green Bean Kale Juice

Ingredients:

1 cup of green beans, chopped

1 cup of fresh kale, torn

1 large apple, cored

1 cup of red leaf lettuce, torn

1 large lime

1 large red bell pepper

1 small ginger root knob, 1-inch

3 oz of water

Preparation:

Wash the green beans and chop into bite-sized pieces. Set aside.

Combine kale and red leaf lettuce in a colander and wash thoroughly under cold running water. Torn with hands and set aside.

Wash the apple and remove the core. Cut into bite-sized pieces and set aside.

Peel the lime and cut lengthwise in half. Set aside.

Wash the red bell pepper and cut in half. Remove the seeds and chop into small pieces. Set aside.

Peel the ginger root knob and set aside.

Now, process green beans, kale, red leaf lettuce, apple, lime, red bell pepper, and ginger root in a juicer.

Transfer to serving glasses and stir in the water. Add some ice and serve immediately.

Nutritional information per serving: Kcal: 194, Protein: 7.1g, Carbs: 52.9g, Fats: 1.7g

24.   Cantaloupe Apple Juice

Ingredients:

2 cups of cantaloupe, chopped

1 large Fuji apple, cored

1 large carrot

1 large orange

1 large lemon

Preparation:

Cut the cantaloupe in half. Scoop out the seeds and flesh. You will need about four large wedges for two cups. Cut and peel them. Chop into chunks and set aside. Reserve the rest of the cantaloupe in a refrigerator.

Wash the apple and remove the core. Cut into bite-sized pieces and set aside.

Peel the orange and lemon. Divide orange into wedges and cut lemon lengthwise in half. Set aside.

Now, process cantaloupe, apple, carrot, orange, and lemon in a juicer.

Transfer to serving glasses and add few ice cubes before serving.

Nutritional information per serving: Kcal: 291, Protein: 6.5g, Carbs: 87.4g, Fats: 1.5g

25.   Asparagus Zucchini Juice

Ingredients:

1 cup of asparagus, trimmed

1 large zucchini

1 cup of collard greens

1 large lemon

2 large leeks

¼ tsp of Himalayan salt

2 oz of water

Preparation:

Wash the asparagus and trim off the woody ends. Cut into small pieces, about 1-inch. Set aside.

Peel the zucchini and cut in half. Scrape out the seeds and cut into chunks. Set aside.

Wash the collard greens thoroughly under cold running water. Drain and torn with hands. Set aside.

Peel the lemon and cut lengthwise in half. Set aside.

Wash the leeks and roughly chop it. Set aside.

Now, combine asparagus, zucchini, collard greens, lemon, and leeks in a juicer and process until juiced.

Transfer to serving glasses and stir in the salt and water.

Refrigerate for 15 minutes before serving.

Nutritional information per serving: Kcal: 171, Protein: 11.2g, Carbs: 47.8g, Fats: 2.1g

26.   Celery Carrot Juice

Ingredients:

2 cups of celery, chopped

3 large carrots

1 large cucumber

1 cup of sweet potatoes, cubed

1 small ginger root knob, 1-inch

Preparation:

Wash the celery and cut into small pieces. Set aside.

Wash the carrots and cucumber. Cut into thick slices and set aside.

Peel the sweet potato and cut into cubes. Fill the measuring cup and reserve the rest for some other juice. Set aside.

Peel the ginger knob and set aside.

Now, process celery, carrots, cucumber, potatoes, and ginger in a juicer.

Transfer to serving glasses and refrigerate for 10 minutes before serving.

Enjoy!

Nutritional information per serving: Kcal: 228, Protein: 7.6g, Carbs: 65.4g, Fats: 1.3g

27.   Pineapple Broccoli Juice

Ingredients:

1 cup of pineapple chunks

1 cup of broccoli

2 cups of green grapes

1 large Granny Smith apple

2 oz of coconut water

1 tsp of honey

Preparation:

Cut the top of a pineapple and peel it using a sharp knife. Cut into small chunks. Reserve the rest of the pineapple in a refrigerator.

Wash the broccoli and cut into small pieces. Set aside.

Place the grapes in a colander and wash under cold running water. Drain and set aside.

Wash the apple and remove the core. Cut into bite-sized pieces and set aside.

Now, combine pineapple chunks, broccoli, grapes, and apple in a juicer and process until juiced.

Transfer to serving glasses and stir in the coconut water and honey. Stir well and add few ice cubes before serving.

Enjoy!

Nutritional information per serving: Kcal: 358, Protein: 5.5g, Carbs: 97.3g, Fats: 1.6g

28.   Squash Pomegranate Juice

Ingredients:

2 cups of butternut squash, chopped

1 cup of pomegranate seeds

1 large lemon

1 large orange

1 cup of celery chopped

2 oz of water

Preparation:

Peel the butternut squash and remove the seeds using a spoon. Cut into small cubes and reserve the rest of the squash for some other recipe. Wrap in a plastic foil and refrigerate.

Cut the top of the pomegranate fruit using a sharp knife. Slice down to each of the white membranes inside of the fruit. Pop the seeds into a medium bowl.

Peel the lemon and orange. Divide orange into wedges and cut lemon lengthwise in half. Set aside.

Wash the celery and chop into small pieces. Set aside.

Now, combine butternut squash, pomegranate seeds, lemon, orange, and celery in a juicer and process until juiced.

Transfer to serving glasses and stir in the water. Add few ice cubes and serve immediately.

Enjoy!

Nutritional information per serving: Kcal: 251, Protein: 7.3g, Carbs: 79g, Fats: 1.8g

29. Collard Greens Carrot Juice

Ingredients:

3 cups of collard greens, torn

2 large carrots

1 medium-sized sweet potato, cubed

1 large cucumber

1 cup of fresh basil, torn

Preparation:

Combine collard greens and basil in a colander. Wash under cold running water and drain. Torn with hands and set aside.

Wash the carrots and cucumber and cut into thick slices. Set aside.

Peel the sweet potato and chop into cubes. Set aside.

Now, process collard greens, carrots, sweet potato, cucumber, and basil in a juicer. Transfer to serving glasses and refigerate for 15 minutes or add some ice and serve immediately.

Nutritional information per serving: Kcal: 201, Protein: 9.3g, Carbs: 57.3g, Fats: 1.5g

30.   Grapefruit Plum Juice

Ingredients:

1 large grapefruit

1 cup of mango, chopped

3 large plums, pitted

1 medium-sized green apple, cored

2 oz of coconut water

A few mint leaves

Preparation:

Peel the grapefruit and divide into wedges. Set aside.

Wash the mango and cut into chunks. Fill the measuring cup and refrigerate the rest for some other juice. Set aside.

Wash the plums and cut in half. Remove the pits and chop into small pieces. Set aside.

Wash the apple and remove the core. Cut into bite-sized pieces and set aside.

Now, process grapefruit, mango, plums, and apple in a juicer. Transfer to serving glasses and stir in the coconut water.

Add few ice cubes and garnish with mint.

Serve immediately.

Nutritional information per serving: Kcal: 211, Protein: 9.3g, Carbs: 59.3g, Fats: 1.5g

31.   Pear Kiwi Juice

Ingredients:

2 large pears, cored

1 large kiwi

1 large cucumber

1 large carrot

2 oz of water

1 tbsp of liquid honey

Preparation:

Wash the pears and remove the core. Cut into bite-sized pieces and set aside.

Peel the kiwi and cut lengthwise in half. Set aside.

Wash the carrot and cucumber and cut into thick slices. Set aside.

Now, combine pears, kiwi, carrot, and cucumber in a juicer and process until juiced. Transfer to serving glasses and add some ice cubes before serving.

Enjoy!

Nutritional information per serving: Kcal: 361, Protein: 5.1g, Carbs: 109g, Fats: 1.5g

32.   Citrus Asparagus Juice

Ingredients:

1 cup of asparagus, trimmed

1 large orange

1 cup of green grapes

1 large lemon

1 large lime

3 oz of water

Preparation:

Wash the asparagus and trim off the woody ends. Cut into 1-inch pieces and set aside.

Peel the orange and divide into wedges. Set aside.

Wash the green grapes under cold running water. Drain water and set aside.

Peel the lemon and lime and cut lengthwise in half. Set aside.

Now, process asparagus, orange, grapes, lemon, and lime in a juicer.

Transfer to serving glasses and stir in the water. Add some ice and serve immediately.

Enjoy!

Nutritional information per serving: Kcal: 361, Protein: 5.1g, Carbs: 109g, Fats: 1.5g

33. Brussels Sprouts Turnip Juice

Ingredients:

2 cups of Brussels sprouts, halved

1 cup of turnip greens, torn

3 large radishes, trimmed

3 large leeks, chopped

1 large cucumber

2 oz of water

Preparation:

Wash the Brussels sprouts and remove the outer layers. Cut in half and set aside.

Wash the turnip greens under cold running water. Drain and torn with hands. Set aside.

Wash the radishes and trim off the green parts. Set aside.

Wash the leeks and cut into bite-sized pieces. Set aside.

Wash the cucumber and cut into thick slices. Set aside.

Now, combine Brussels sprouts, turnip greens, radishes, leeks, and cucumber in a juicer and process until juiced. Transfer to serving glasses and stir in the water.

Refrigerate for 10 minutes before serving.

Nutritional information per serving: Kcal: 247, Protein: 12.9g, Carbs: 69.3g, Fats: 1.8g

34.   Purple Cabbage Mango Juice

Ingredients:

2 large Fuji apples, cored

1 cup of purple cabbage, torn

1 cup of mango, chopped

1 cup of fresh basil, torn

1 small carrot

¼ tsp of ginger, ground

Preparation:

Wash the apples and remove the core. Cut into bite-sized pieces and set aside.

Combine cabbage and basil in a colander. Wash thoroughly under cold running water and torn with hands. Set aside.

Wash the mango and cut into small chunks. Fill the measuring cup and reserve the rest for some other juice. Set aside.

Wash the carrot and cut into thick slices. Set aside.

Now, process apples, purple cabbage, mango, basil, and carrots in a juicer. Transfer to serving glasses and stir in ginger.

Refrigerate for about 10-15 minutes before serving.

Nutritional information per serving: Kcal: 319, Protein: 5.6g, Carbs: 92.7g, Fats: 1.8g

35.   Tomato Cauliflower Juice

Ingredients:

2 medium-sized tomatoes

1 large red bell pepper, chopped

1 cup of cauliflower

1 large lime

3 oz of water

1 tsp of fresh rosemary, finely chopped

Preparation:

Wash the tomatoes and place them in a bowl. Cut into quarters and reserve the juice while cutting. Set aside.

Wash the bell pepper and cut in half. Remove the seeds and chop into small slices. Set aside.

Trim off the outer leaves of cauliflower. Wash it and cut into small pieces. Reserve the rest in the refrigerator.

Peel the lime and cut lengthwise in half. Set aside.

Now, combine tomatoes, red bell pepper, cauliflower, and lime in a juicer and process until juiced.

Transfer to serving glasses and stir in the reserved tomato juice and water. Sprinkle with fresh rosemary and refrigerate for 10 minutes before serving.

Enjoy!

Nutritional information per serving: Kcal: 98, Protein: 6g, Carbs: 28.5g, Fats: 1.3g

36.   Blueberry Banana Juice

Ingredients:

2 cups of blueberries

1 large banana

1 small Golden Delicious apple, cored

1 large cucumber

2 oz of water

Preparation:

Place the blueberries in a colander and wash under cold running water. Drain and set aside.

Peel the banana and cut into small chunks. Set aside.

Wash the apple and remove the core. Cut into bite-sized pieces and set aside.

Wash the cucumber and cut into thick slices. Set aside.

Now, process blueberries, banana, apple, and cucumber in a juicer. Transfer to serving glasses and add some ice before serving.

Enjoy!

Nutritional information per serving: Kcal: 348, Protein: 6g, Carbs: 102g, Fats: 1.9g

37.   Romaine Lettuce Artichoke Juice

Ingredients:

3 cups of Romaine lettuce

1 cup of spinach, torn

1 medium-sized artichoke

1 large Honeydew melon wedge

1 small green apple, cored

2 large carrots

2 oz of water

Preparation:

Wash the lettuce and spinach thoroughly under cold running water and set aside.

Trim off the outer leaves of the artichoke using a sharp knife. Cut into small pieces and set aside.

Cut the honeydew melon lengthwise in half. Scoop out the seeds using a spoon. Cut one large wedge and peel them. Cut into small chunks and fill the measuring cup. Wrap the rest of the melon in a plastic foil and refrigerate.

Wash the apple and remove the core. Cut into bite-sized pieces and set aside.

Wash the carrots and cut into thick slices. Set aside.

Now, combine lettuce, artichoke, honeydew melon, apple, and carrots in a juicer and process until juiced. Transfer to serving glasses and stir in the water.

Add some ice and serve immediately.

Nutritional information per serving: Kcal: 213, Protein: 9.6g, Carbs: 67.1g, Fats: 1.5g

38.   Cantaloupe Squash Juice

Ingredients:

2 cups of cantaloupe

1 cup of crookneck squash, chopped

1 cup of raspberries

1 large apricot

1 large kiwi

Preparation:

Cut the cantaloupe in half. Scoop out the seeds and flesh. Cut two wedges and peel them. Chop into chunks and set aside. Reserve the rest of the cantaloupe in a refrigerator.

Wash the crookneck squash and cut in half. Scoop out the seeds using a spoon. Cut into small chunks and set aside. Reserve the rest for another juice.

Wash the raspberries under cold running water and set aside.

Wash the apricot and cut in half. Remove the pit and cut into chunks. Set aside.

Peel the kiwi and cut lengthwise in half. Set aside.

Now, process cantaloupe, crookneck squash, raspberries, apricots, and kiwi in a juicer.

Transfer to serving glasses and add some ice before serving.

Enjoy!

Nutritional information per serving: Kcal: 193, Protein: 6.6g, Carbs: 59.1g, Fats: 2.3g

39.   Parsnip Pepper Juice

Ingredients:

2 cups of parsnips

1 large green bell pepper

1 cup of Swiss chard, torn

1 large cucumber

1 ginger root knob, 1-inch

2 oz of water

Preparation:

Wash the parsnips and trim off the green parts. Cut into bite-sized pieces and set aside.

Wash the bell pepper and cut into half. Remove the seeds and cut into small slices. Set aside.

Wash the Swiss chard thoroughly and torn with hands. Set aside.

Peel the ginger and set aside.

Now, process parsnips, bell pepper, Swiss chard, cucumber, and ginger knob in a juicer.

Transfer to serving glasses and stir in the water.

Add some ice and serve immediately.

Enjoy!

Nutritional information per serving: Kcal: 219, Protein: 7.3g, Carbs: 68.8g, Fats: 1.5g

40.   Peach Cranberry Juice

Ingredients:

1 large peach

1 cup of cranberries

2 small Granny Smith apples

1 cup of grapes

2 oz of water

Preparation:

Wash the peach and cut in half. Remove the pit and cut into chunks. Set aside.

Wash the cranberries and grapes under cold running water and set aside.

Wash the apples and remove the core. Cut into bite-sized pieces and set aside.

Now, combine peach, cranberries, apples, and grapes in a juicer and process until juiced. Transfer to serving glasses and add some ice.

Serve immediately.

Nutritional information per serving: Kcal: 284, Protein: 2.8g, Carbs: 85g, Fats: 1.4g

41.   Papaya Grapefruit Juice

Ingredients:

1 cup of papaya, chopped

1 large grapefruit

1 large cucumber

1 small green apple

2 oz of coconut water

Preparation:

Peel the papaya and cut lengthwise in half. Scoop out the black seeds and flesh using a spoon. Cut into small chunks and fill the measuring cup. Reserve the rest for some other juice. Set aside.

Peel the grapefruit and divide into wedges. Set aside.

Wash the cucumber and cut into thick slices. Set aside.

Wash the apple and remove the core. Cut into bite-sized pieces and set aside.

Now, process papaya, grapefruit, cucumber, and apple in a juicer. Transfer to serving glasses and stir in the coconut water.

Add few ice cubes and serve immediately.

Nutritional information per serving: Kcal: 246, Protein: 5.1g, Carbs: 72.4g, Fats: 1.3g

42.   Pomegranate Strawberry Juice

Ingredients:

1 cup of pomegranate seeds

1 cup of strawberries

1 large green apple

1 large orange

A handful of spinach

2 oz of water

Preparation:

Cut the top of the pomegranate fruit using a sharp knife. Slice down to each of the white membranes inside of the fruit. Pop the seeds into a medium bowl.

Wash the strawberries and cut in half. Set aside.

Wash the apple and remove the core. Cut into bite-sized pieces and set aside.

Wash the spinach thoroughly and torn with hands. Set aside.

Peel the orange and divide into wedges. Set aside.

Now, process pomegranate seeds, strawberries, apple, spinach, and orange in a juicer. Transfer to serving glasses and stir in the water.

Refrigerate for 15 minutes before serving.

Nutritional information per serving: Kcal: 266, Protein: 6.1g, Carbs: 80.8g, Fats: 2.2g

43.   Green Bean Zucchini Juice

Ingredients:

1 cup of green beans, chopped

1 large zucchini, chopped

1 cup of sweet potatoes

1 large lemon

¼ tsp of Himalayan salt

2 oz of water

Preparation:

Wash the green beans and cut into 1-inch pieces. Set aside.

Peel the zucchini and cut in half. Scoop out the seeds and cut into chunks. Set aside.

Peel the sweet potatoes and cut into small cubes. Fill the measuring cup and reserve the rest for some other juice. Set aside.

Peel the lemon and cut lengthwise in half. Set aside.

Now, process green beans, zucchini, sweet potatoes, and lemon in a juicer and stir in the water.

Add some ice or refrigerate before serving.

Enjoy!

Nutritional information per serving: Kcal: 171, Protein: 7.6g, Carbs: 46g, Fats: 1.3g

44.　　Kale Cucumber Juice

Ingredients:

3 cups of fresh kale, torn

1 large cucumber

1 large plum

1 small green apple, cored

1 tbsp of honey

2 oz of water

Preparation:

Wash the kale thoroughly under cold running water. Drain and set aside.

Wash the cucumber and cut into thick slices. Set aside.

Wash the plum and cut in half. Remove the pit and cut into small pieces. Set aside.

Wash the apple and remove the core. Cut into bite-sized pieces and set aside.

Now, combine kale, cucumber, plum, and apple in a juicer and process until juiced. Transfer to serving glasses and stir in the honey and water.

Enjoy!

Nutritional information per serving: Kcal: 262, Protein: 11.6g, Carbs: 72.6g, Fats: 2.6g

45.   Mango Beet Juice

Ingredients:

1 cup of mango, chopped

3 large beets, trimmed

1 small apple, cored

1 cup of broccoli

3 oz of coconut water

Preparation:

Wash the mango and cut into chunks. Fill the measuring cup and reserve the rest for some other juice. Set aside.

Wash the beets and trim off the green parts. Cut into small pieces and set aside.

Wash the apple and remove the core. Cut into bite-sized pieces and set aside.

Wash the broccoli and cut into small pieces. Set aside.

Now, combine mango, beets, apple, and broccoli in a juicer and process until juiced.

Transfer to serving glasses and add some ice before serving.

Enjoy!

Nutritional information per serving: Kcal: 260, Protein: 8.2g, Carbs: 71.8g, Fats: 1.6g

46.   Cherry Apple Juice

Ingredients:

1 cup of cherries

1 small apple, cored

1 large carrot

1 large orange

1 large lemon

2 oz of water

Preparation:

Wash the cherries thoroughly and cut in half. Remove the pits and set aside.

Wash the apple and remove the core. Cut into bite-sized pieces and set aside.

Wash the carrot and cut into thick slices. Set aside.

Peel the lemon and orange. Cut lemon lengthwise in half and divide orange into wedges. Set aside.

Now, combine cherries, apple, carrot, lemon, and orange in a juicer and process until juiced. Transfer to serving glasses and add some ice before serving.

Enjoy!

Nutritional information per serving: Kcal: 253, Protein: 5.3g, Carbs: 78.2g, Fats: 1.1g

ADDITIONAL TITLES FROM THIS AUTHOR

70 Effective Meal Recipes to Prevent and Solve Being Overweight: Burn Fat Fast by Using Proper Dieting and Smart Nutrition

By

Joe Correa CSN

48 Acne Solving Meal Recipes: The Fast and Natural Path to Fixing Your Acne Problems in Less Than 10 Days!

By

Joe Correa CSN

41 Alzheimer's Preventing Meal Recipes: Reduce or Eliminate Your Alzheimer's Condition in 30 Days or Less!

By

Joe Correa CSN

70 Effective Breast Cancer Meal Recipes: Prevent and Fight Breast Cancer with Smart Nutrition and Powerful Foods

By

Joe Correa CSN

CPSIA information can be obtained
at www.ICGtesting.com
Printed in the USA
BVOW08s1051090118
504830BV00001B/107/P